TRANSIT

"A Brief Journey of Self-Discovery, Hope, and New Beginnings "

Kenneth P. Griffin

Copyright © 2023 by Kenneth P. Griffin

All rights reserved. No part of this book may be reproduced in any form or by any electronic or mechanical means, including information storage and retrieval systems, without written permission from the author, except for the use of brief quotations in a book review.

This book is a work of nonfiction. The names, characters, places, and incidents are products of the author's imagination or have been used fictitiously. Any resemblance to actual persons, living or dead, events, or locales is entirely coincidental.

TABLE OF CONTENTS

INTRODUCTION

Transit generally refers to the movement or transit of people or objects from one location to another. However, in this study, we will be looking at it from an unusual or distinctive perspective. Believe it or not, we are on a journey as humans. It is why humans grow old and die. On the other hand, life and everything in it follow this motion trend. As is well known, the Earth and everything in it is constantly spinning. God designed it that way.

Hence, focusing on humans and our daily lives, it will be an anomaly for a person to remain static in terms of growth in all aspects of life. We should advance spiritually, mentally, financially, and otherwise, according to God's plan. Yet, this development must be looked at through your moral lens because you want to ensure your "peace of mind" is intact as you progress through these different phases.

Are you going through any emotional, relationship, financial, or mental struggles? It's time to "transit" to a better location in every element of your life.

You can bring about the change you desire; all you need is to tap into the virtues you possess. Happily, it is exactly what the life-changing information in this book is for. The keys in this book will bring out a side of you that you never knew existed. You hold an invaluable piece in your hands.

I encourage you to read with an open mind and heart since only then will this pearl benefit you.

Happy reading.

CHAPTER ONE

BECOME SELF-AWARE

Self-awareness involves having a sense of one's identity, feelings, thoughts, and behaviors and being able to reflect on these things consciously. It involves clearly understanding who you are and how you fit into the world around you. It is taking cognizance of your abilities and everything you have been blessed with. Today's world is filled with people who don't know who they are. As a result, their lives tend to take a different and unanticipated trajectory, and they seem unable to do anything about it.

Many people need to learn what their abilities are, what they can and cannot do, their strengths, and their limitations. And this is largely because they need to be self- aware. Yes, self-awareness needs to be improved on many fronts. And until a person understands who he is, I'm sorry, but such a person will hardly impact his environment. That is why if you must make massive strides in your life, achieving self -awareness is key. If you don't like your life's direction, it is time for you to embark on this journey consciously.

There are a few different but practical ways that individuals can work on developing their self-awareness. Here are a few tips.

• **Practice Seeing Yourself the Way God sees you**: This is doubtlessly the most important means of achieving self-awareness. This is the primary way to reach an essential point in self-awareness. As the term states, self-awareness simply is KNOWING oneself. The Bible tells us in Genesis 1:26 that we are made in the image and Likeness of God. This connotes that man is a replica of the Almighty God. But you can only realize this when you start seeing yourself as God sees you. And the way to do this is to be well acquainted with the word of God.

It means you must give attention to the word of God as often as possible. This is strongly encouraged because, as you give time to the word, your thoughts start aligning with God's thoughts for you. For instance, if God sees you as a successful person (and He surely does) and you, on the other hand, see yourself as a failure, you will invariably hinder that good thought of God for you from manifesting.

According to 3 John 1:2, "Beloved, I wish above all things that thou mayest prosper and be in health, even as thy soul prospers." This is why your acquaintance with the knowledge of God's word is non-negotiable. It must become your "best friend." Some people think that becoming self-aware is a natural part of growing up and maturing, while others think it is something we are born with and can't change.

While that may be true to an extent, a quicker route to this vast Highland is what we have just looked at. I am bold enough to declare that any man's success, regardless of who he is, begins the moment he starts to see himself the way God sees him. That is the turning point.

Now, how does this translate into you becoming a better person? The fact that you are reading this book shows how much you want to change. Hence, this prescription is vital for the change you anticipate. It would be beneficial if you deliberately practiced obeying the command. That is the primary means by which you can become the person you want to be. Will it be easy? No. But will it be worth it in the long run? A gigantic YES.

- **Journaling**: Recording your thoughts and feelings in a journal can help you reflect on your experiences and gain insight into your mind.

- **Therapy**: Engaging with a therapist or counselor can provide a safe and supportive setting to explore your thoughts, feelings, and actions.

- **Get feedback from others**: Getting feedback from those familiar with you might help you gain a new perspective on yourself and your activities.

- **Practice self-reflection**: thinking about your experiences, habits, and emotions can help you better understand yourself. Some people can access their depth or innermost thoughts when they are still. For others who are too busy working. Others when they are walking quickly. Others may be in a huge group listening to someone speak, such as at a conference, seminar, or even a church service (this works a lot for me). As a result, "identifying your stance" is critical in discovering oneself.

- **Be willing to learn about yourself**: It's critical to discover new things about yourself, including your ideas, feelings, and habits. This could include trying new things, being open to new experiences, and being willing to question your assumptions and views.

● Pay attention to your emotions: Your emotions can provide a wealth of information about yourself and your needs. Paying attention to your emotions and attempting to comprehend their causes and triggers might assist you in being more self-aware.

● Practicing self-compassion entails treating yourself with the same kindness, care, and understanding that you would extend to a good friend. Self-compassion can help you accept your imperfections and mistakes, leading to better self-awareness.

● Seek out new experiences: Experimenting with new things and being exposed to new situations can help you learn more about yourself and your interests, values, and abilities.

● Accept responsibility for your acts and their repercussions: Taking responsibility for your actions and their consequences is important to developing self-awareness. It can assist you in better understanding the impact of your actions on people and the world around you, allowing you to make better decisions in the future.

What are the benefits of being self-aware?

Self-awareness has various advantages. The greater our self-awareness, the better we can control our emotions. We can adjust our behavior when we recognize our strengths and weaknesses.

On the road to success, having self-awareness and self-reflection helps us comprehend the impact of our actions on others. It teaches us to be more considerate of others and live more ethically. It can also help us improve our spiritual discernment in our daily lives.

Self-awareness allows us to grow closer to God and become the best versions of ourselves, just as God intended. When you increase your self-awareness, you will have more creativity, self-esteem, and self-acceptance. Self-aware people are more likely to become stronger leaders on the job and spiritually. They are also more likely to inspire followers' trust and collaboration.

More self-acceptance and less severe self-judgment should be the goal of self-awareness. Remember that self-awareness is a process that takes time and effort to understand and be aware of yourself completely. Yet, with effort and commitment, you may develop your self-awareness and better understand who you are.

CHAPTER TWO

DESIRE A CHANGE, AND EFFECT IT

What is your Desire? It is possible to desire true love and yet request fleeting Pleasures. If you will see the change you desire, your heart and mind must be aligned. They must be in sync. Your entire being must be in unity for your desires to manifest quickly. Have you seen a drug addict? Most of the time, they will do anything to satisfy their urge, regardless of the consequences. That is how you must desire a change in your life. If you must transit to where you envisage, your Desire for that positive change must be overwhelming.

How badly do you want things to change? Let me show you a verse in psalm 145:15 -16, "The eyes of all wait upon you, and you give them their meat in due season. you open your hand, and satisfies the desire of every living thing". Did you see that? The scriptures say even God satisfies your Desire.

So, what if a person has no desire? It means there is nothing God can do for that person. People are walking about the streets complaining about this or that. Yet such people, when asked about what they want, are so vague about their desires. Don't be like that. Know what you want. Know your desires.

A healthy person wants things and situations to be better than they are. If you must make progress, you must fuel your Desire for change.

The Key to Making Your Dreams a Reality

• Identify what you want to change: It is critical to be clear about what to change since this will help you design a strategy to make the change happen. This is vital since you do not want to outrun the wind at any cost. You want to be as precise as possible in your actions. It is critical to hitting the nail on the head to see the desired change.

• Create a strategy: Once you've decided what to change, the next step is to think about the steps required to bring about the desired change. Transform your long-term goal into a series of small, more manageable steps.

- **Start moving**: To effect the desired change, you must start moving and take action. Even though the task is difficult, it is necessary to retain concentration and resolve.

- **Leave your comfort zone**: To make big changes, you may need to leave your comfort zone from time to time. This could be terrifying, but it could also be wonderful and rewarding.

- **Get assistance if necessary**: making changes may be easier if you have the support of others. Tell your loved ones and friends about your plans, and ask for their support and encouragement, but only if you are convinced that they will see the new obligations positively. After all, it is best to go alone rather than with someone who does not believe in one's talents. Amos 3:3, Can two persons walk together unless they agree?

- **Make your desires a reality by rehearsing them:** This statement captures the essence of the chapter. Due to the Law of Attraction, your words are one of the most powerful tools since you can speak things into existence using them.

According to the law of Attraction, also known as the law of Manifestation, you attract into your life whatever you focus on in your thoughts. Furthermore, the words that come out of your mouth are a direct reflection of the thoughts that are running through your mind.

To use the Law of Attraction to bring things into existence, you must ensure that your thoughts and words align with what you want.

If you want to create a circumstance in which you have abundant financial resources, make sure that the focus of your conversations is on how easy it is to get money rather than how difficult it is to generate money.

If you want to attract a love partner into your life, make sure that the focus of your conversations is on how much fun going on dates is rather than how tough it is to locate "the one."

You can't have your heart's Desire while also being able to speak critically about it. Whatever issue you focus on most in your interactions, whether good or terrible, will become a reality in your life.

Can I manifest my desires merely by voicing them? Yes. You can talk your desires into being. Everything that happens to you in life is a direct outcome of your thinking. And how you express yourself vocally reflects how you think. You can only create what you think about and talk about in your thoughts and conversations.

When you focus on and talk about the things you don't want, those things will come into your life. Whatever your primary focus is, you attract more of it into your life. You bring into being whatever you focus the majority of your attention on.

The following steps are below to learn how to apply the Law of Attraction to manifest your desires simply by speaking them into existence.

a. You Should Only Talk About Things That Interest You

The first step in using the Law of Attraction to bring things into existence is limiting your discourse to only what you wish. You will experience a dramatic shift as a result of this. According to Genesis 1:3, the Earth was wrapped in darkness; however, God did not focus on the circumstance but on what He intended, so He proceeded to create light.

In other words, God focused on what He wished rather than the situation. The verse ends with the phrase, "And there was light." God's working is described in Romans 4:17, where he "calls those things which are not as though they existed." God operates in this manner. This is how He desires us to live every day.

Unfortunately, many people are raised with the mindset of focusing on things that aren't working or that they don't want. We prefer to summon the things we don't want rather than the things we do want.

Because we constantly say things like, "I am tired, broke, and I dislike my job," the Law of Attraction drives us to attract undesirable circumstances due to the words we use. The good news is that the Law of Attraction also attracts things into our lives that we desire to happen.

The most crucial thing for you to do now is to shift your internal dialogue to things that are going well in your life or that you want to create. My preferred way for redirecting your speech toward your goals is to use affirmations. You may raise your vibration by repeating these affirmations about yourself.

b. Belief in what you're saying.

The second stage in using the Law of Attraction to bring things into existence through the power of your words is to believe in what you say. Your affirmations should not be so far out of reach that you can't force yourself to believe in them.

For example, you may tell yourself, "I want to be a millionaire by tomorrow," yet you may not achieve that goal because you recognize, on some level, that it is unrealistic. When you speak your affirmations, make sure they resonate with you and that even the most primal portions of your body can feel the resonance of what you're saying.

Make changes to your affirmations until you can say that you completely believe what you're saying. Instead of "I am going to materialize a million dollars tomorrow," try rephrasing your affirmation to say something like, "I am happy to find new ways of producing money," or "I am feeling hopeful about my financial future."

How long does it take until you notice the desired change?

Starting the process of speaking things into existence can take anywhere from a few days to a few weeks. The time it takes to finish depends on how well your ideas are aligned with the desired goal.

You will only succeed in making your wish tangible if you constantly focus on the possibility of doing so. You can't focus on the fact that you don't already have what you want while bringing it into being.

Most of your ideas must be consistent with the conviction that you can achieve your goals and receive what you desire. No self- criticism, self-doubt, or whining about how difficult it is to achieve what you desire should be tolerated.

You will reach your goals as long as you are confident that you can do so. Is it always possible to "speak things into existence" (also known as "create reality")? Yes. Just speaking anything into existence will always bring it to pass.

Sometimes, it is likely that the event will unfold much better than you anticipated. For example, instead of imagining yourself in a new position at a certain organization, you may envision yourself starting your own internet business. This is a more particular embodiment of what you desire. Instead of attempting to form a love connection with a certain person, you may go to a coffee shop and have a conversation with a stranger.

As a result, you mustn't impose any constraints on how you feel your Manifestation will occur. Always keep an open mind to the possibility of creative solutions. Keep your alignment to create what you desire, but let go of the details of how this will happen.

● **Be patient**: adjusting to change takes time, so remember to be patient and give yourself lots of time.

● **Remember to celebrate your triumphs** as you get closer to your goals, and do so as you progress toward those goals. This can help you keep your motivation up and allow you to keep making progress.

Remember that change does not happen overnight. Although it will take time and effort, remember the adage that "nothing good comes easy."

CHAPTER THREE

HAVE FAITH IN YOURSELF

Believing in yourself and your ability is important to your success and achievement of your goals. It entails believing in your talents and trusting your judgment to pick the best action. When you believe in yourself, you are more inclined to take risks and try new things, which can benefit your personal development and education.

As a result, you will become more resilient and better able to recover from failures, making it simpler to overcome issues and setbacks. Remember that you are not perfect and that mistakes are normal. What is most essential is to learn from your mistakes and keep moving forward. If you believe in your identity and talents, you will be well on your way to doing whatever you set out to do.

When it comes to believing in yourself, the following are some more considerations to consider:

- **Make it a point to practice self-acceptance**. It is critical to be kind to yourself and accept who you are, even if you are aware of areas of your personality that could use improvement. Although we all have defects, we must recognize and respect the characteristics that distinguish us and our unique talents.

• **Give yourself the attention and care you deserve** to ensure your physical, emotional, and mental well-being. When you have a healthy perspective on yourself and your life, you will be better positioned to believe in your skills and make sound judgments.

• **Establish your goals and strive toward obtaining them.** Understanding where you want to go and what you want to achieve can help you focus your efforts and give you a sense of purpose. When you progress toward your goals and see that you are succeeding, your confidence in your ability to succeed grows.

• **Surround yourself with people who have faith** in you and want you to succeed. Being surrounded by individuals who believe in you and support your ambitions may be a fantastic source of motivation and encouragement. Pick happy and motivating people, and avoid those who are constantly finding fault or criticizing others.

Because the people we spend our time with greatly influence our lives, we must fill our spheres of influence with people who benefit us. Being around people who are upbeat, supportive, and encouraging might make us happier, more confident, and more motivated.

Spending time with negative or toxic people, on the other hand, can drain our energy, make us feel sad, and even be harmful to our mental and emotional well-being. It is critical to ensure that you are surrounded by positive influences which support your objectives and values by taking the time to analyze the relationships in your life and ensuring that positive influences surround you.

Why it's critical to surround yourself with positive and supportive people

Consider the following additional concepts about the importance of surrounding yourself with the right company:

• Surrounding oneself with enthusiastic and optimistic people may assist you in maintaining a positive attitude and outlook on life.

• Being surrounded by caring and supportive friends and family can help you feel less isolated, which is especially crucial during difficult times.

• Establishing positive relationships with others can boost your confidence, self-esteem, and self-worth.

• Spending time with negative or poisonous people, on the other hand, can depress you and sap your vigor. It's also probable that it'll be bad for your mental and emotional well-being.

• Surrounding yourself with people who share your objectives and beliefs will help to keep you motivated and on track to attain the goals you've set for yourself.

• Remember that you can choose who works in your firm. If you notice that a certain person or group of people is not positively impacting your life, it may be necessary to distance yourself from them or minimize the amount of time you spend with them.

BE POSITIVE

Mark 9:23, Jesus responded to him by saying, "If you can believe, you will see that all things are possible for you who believe."

Everything we have discussed up until this point revolves around these two words: BE POSITIVE. The value of a positive mindset cannot be overstated. It would help if you remembered this as you go on this road to becoming a better version of yourself. It would help if you did not let the fact that you will probably fail sometimes prevent you from following through on your decision and efforts to become a better version of yourself.

No athlete becomes a professional overnight. It usually takes some time to get there. The capacity to maintain an optimistic outlook, on the other hand, is what musters that strength and courage. Remember that having faith in oneself is a process that takes time. If you are patient with yourself and continue striving toward the goals you have set for yourself, you will progress and succeed in your life.

You should be aware that sometimes opposition might come from people you least expect it to come from, but that's just how life works. People only want to be associated with successful people; therefore, you need to be tenacious in pursuing new opportunities. I'll see you at the top!

www.ingramcontent.com/pod-product-compliance
Lightning Source LLC
Chambersburg PA
CBHW051430250726
48656CB00020B/2322